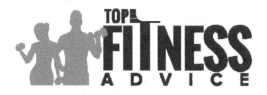

LIFE SAVING FOODS

How You Can Benefit From 15 Foods That Make You Healthier, More Energized, & Have A Longer Life

Bonus: 50 Quick & Easy Life Saving Food Recipes!

LINDA WESTWOOD

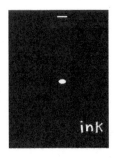

First published in 2017 by Venture Ink Publishing

Copyright © Top Fitness Advice 2019

For more information about the contents of this book or questions to the author, please contact Linda Westwood at linda@topfitnessadvice.com

Disclaimer

This book provides wellness management information in an informative and educational manner only, with information that is general in nature and that is not specific to you, the reader. The contents of this book are intended to assist you and other readers in your personal wellness efforts. Consult your physician regarding the applicability of any information provided in this book to you.

Nothing in this book should be construed as personal advice or diagnosis, and must not be used in this manner. The information provided about conditions is general in nature. This information does not cover all possible uses, actions, precautions, side-effects, or interactions of medicines, or medical procedures. The information in this book should not be considered as complete and does not cover all diseases, ailments, physical conditions, or their treatment.

You should consult with your physician before beginning any exercise, weight loss, or health care program. This book should not be used in place of a call or visit to a competent health-care professional. You should consult a health care professional before adopting any of the suggestions in this book or before drawing inferences from it.

Any decision regarding treatment and medication for your condition should be made with the advice and consultation of a qualified health care professional. If you have, or suspect you have, a health-care problem, then you should immediately contact a qualified health care professional for treatment.

No Warranties: The author and publisher don't guarantee or warrant the quality, accuracy, completeness, timeliness, appropriateness or suitability of the information in this book, or of any product or services referenced in this book.

The information in this book is provided on an "as is" basis and the author and publisher make no representations or warranties of any kind with respect to this information. This book may contain inaccuracies, typographical errors, or other errors.

Table of Contents

Would you prefer to listen to my book, rather than read it?

Download the audiobook version for free!

If you go to the special link below and sign up to Audible as a new customer, you can get the audiobook version of my book completely free.

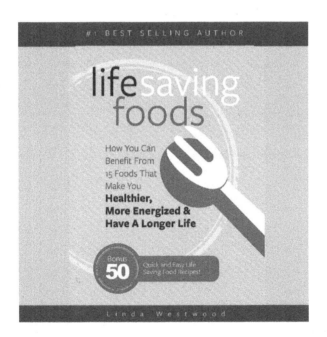

Go here to get your audiobook version for free:

TopFitnessAdvice.com/go/LifeFoods

Introduction

If you've picked up this book, the chances are that you are striving towards a healthier lifestyle. That could be through exercise alone, it could be through changing your diet, or it could be the best possible route – a combination of both.

There are certain foods which we should all be getting our daily quota of, because these are not only truly delicious, cost effective, and add flavour to sometimes mundane dishes, but they are also packed with all the vitamins and minerals you need for overall health and wellbeing. If you don't eat these foods, you're going to be lacking in the things you need to keep you fit and strong.

This book is designed to help people like you, those who want to become healthier, but don't really know where to start. The good news? We're going to make it really simple for you, and by the end of reading, you'll know all you need to embark on a heathier food. We're also going to give you 50 bonus recipes to get you into the kitchen and rustling up some fantastic dishes to enjoy.

Now, the name of the book should give you some clue as the subject matter at hand. There are certain foods which can save your life. Literally! These foods are anti-oxidant rich, mineral rich, vitamin rich, and basically are bright, colourful, and taste delicious all at the same time. There used to be the old adage of 'five a day' for your fresh fruit and vegetables, but these days that number has increased.

This is because these foods are easy to incorporate into your diet, and the more you get, the better your overall health and wellbeing will be. Of course, at this point, you will have no idea what those foods are, but by the end of this book you will be a super-whizz on the foods that can boost your health and have you jumping through hoops in no time!

So, what can you expect to get out of this book?

We are going to talk about health, we're going to tell you what you should be doing, what you should be avoiding, and why it's all totally worthwhile. We're also going to give you those 50 recipes we talked about, and these are all easy to make, the ingredients are readily available and cost effective, and the entire family will be licking their lips by the end of their serving.

We're also going to talk a little about exercise, and why incorporating exercise into your daily routine can give you an even bigger boost.

First things first however, let's move onto our first chapter and explore exactly what health is, and what you can do to boost yours.

Chapter 1

Health & Wellness 101

Welcome to the beginning of your journey towards total health and wellbeing! This chapter is going to give you the background information you need, arming you with important facts to push yourself towards a healthier future.

First of all however, we need to know what health and wellness is, and we need to know exactly why it is so important. What is health? What is wellness? Why do we need to avoid certain things?

Let's explore in more detail.

What is Health and Wellness?

This might sound like a ridiculous question, but to give a thorough overview, you need to know the basics! Health is about your body having all the vitamins, minerals, and fuel it needs to run in the most effective way possible. If you don't give your body what it needs, then it is not going to be able to do its job, and you are going to start having symptoms of problems.

Example, if you don't drink enough water, your body becomes dehydrated, and that shows itself in tiredness, headaches, lack of energy, dry skin and lips etc. This is just one example, and a simple one at that, but it displays the issue very clearly.

Everyone has the odd unhealthy habit, and these aren't the biggest problem in the world provided you exercise moderation within them. For instance, if you like the odd glass of wine, there is no harm in that provided that the odd glass doesn't turn into the odd bottle, or the odd glass doesn't turn into every night. A little bit of what we like is a good thing, because it helps us keep a balance in our lives between health and happiness.

Of course, that's not to say that you can't be ultra-happy when you're being healthy, because there are some fantastic foods and recipes out there, which are even tastier than those things which are 'bad' for you!

Generally speaking, you are considered to be doing your bit for your overall health and wellbeing if you are doing the following things:

- Exercising regularly

- Not smoking, or working to cut down

- Only consuming alcohol in moderation, occasionally

- Making sure your diet is varied and free of too much saturated fat

- If you are getting a variation of vitamins and minerals, through fresh fruit and vegetables every single day

- You watch the amount of sugar you eat every day

- You have regular check-ups with your doctor, and you get anything unusual checked out straight away

- You vary your diet to avoid boredom

- You wear sun-cream during the summer and when out in direct sunlight for long periods of time

- You brush your teeth every day

- You keep up with your personal hygiene

Most of these you probably tick off, such as the personal hygiene, brushing teeth, getting unusual things checked out with the doctor, but do you meet the criteria of the other things? Do you exercise regularly? Do you eat plenty of fresh fruit and vegetables? Do you keep your diet varied to give your body all the nutrition it needs?

Not that many people can nod along to that and be honest about it.

The good news is that the situation is reversible.

Social Pressures and Their Impact on Our Health and Wellness

Today we have other pressures aside from wanting to look and feel good, because we have the added extra of social media and social pressures. These days we have an overwhelming tendency to compare ourselves to others, and the access to those whom we compare ourselves with is huge now that we can see the lives of everyone else right from our smartphone.

If you're a little overweight, you begin to compare yourself to someone's Facebook picture of them on a beach looking amazing. Of course, that photo has probably been Instagrammed and filtered to within an inch of its life, but you don't have solid proof of that, and your mind isn't going down that route – you are thinking that they look amazing and you don't, and then the downward spiral of upset and paranoia begins.

There are too many negative roads which lead off a poor body confidence level, e.g. eating disorders, body dysmorphia, depression, and anxiety, to name just a few.

The choice to be healthy will help you avoid these pitfalls, because you are targeting your mind at the important things in life – giving your body the fuel, vitamins, and minerals it needs to function properly, and this has a hugely positive effect on not only your physical body, but your mind and your soul also. It sounds cliché, but it's a truth.

We are also bombarded with images of what we said to be 'perfection', but how decided what perfection is? Who said that being slim is perfect? Who said that having a larger breast size is perfect? Who said that having muscles is perfect?

We are all individual, and provided you are a healthy weight for your height, your BMI is within the normal range (body mass index), and you are happy with yourself, that is really all that matters. Having said that, social media and society itself does us no favours in terms of helping us feel about ourselves, when there really is no reason to do so.

The answer? You could go on a social media diet for a while and block out those images whilst you get to work on your overall health and wellbeing, before drip feeding it back into your life if you want to; you could even avoid everything socially annoying to you and your body shape, but that would be rather difficult to do.

No, the best option is to change your mindset towards being comfortable in your own skin, and getting to work on your body, your health, and making sure you give your system everything it needs to do its great work – your body performs miracles every single day!

Small Changes Make a Huge Difference

In terms of making changes to your lifestyle, this doesn't have to be massive, drastic changes at all at once, because smaller changes can be just as effective over a period of time. You may even find that if you make too many big changes, your body rebels against it all and wonders what on earth is going on. This means you're going to get side effects which may be difficult to cope with, sending you back to your old unhealthy ways.

The best course of action here is to take baby steps. Assess your lifestyle as it is currently and identify what changes you need to make – write a list if you need to.

From there, prioritise those changes; if you need to stop smoking, make that your priority, before moving onto the next one, and if you need to begin exercising, start incorporating that into your week in a slow manner, before building it up gradually. Over time these changes will have a very cumulative effect, and you will see results in a much bigger and more sustainable way as a result.

Make Changes for You, and You Alone!

Of course, the most important thing to note here is the reason why you are making these lifestyle changes. There is only one acceptable answer to the question – the answer is that you are doing it for you, and you alone. You cannot make these changes for anyone else, because once their motivation or interests shifts, your desire to continue with your healthier lifestyle is going to wane, and you'll be back to square one.

Making a commitment to your overall health is one of the biggest and most rewarding changes you will make in your life, so make sure you are basing it on the right motivation, and not for some other reason.

Many people change their lives as revenge on someone else, e.g. after a break up with an ex, for example, and whilst that is a good motivation to get started, the baseline reason has to be because you want to do it for your own future – there is no problem with having a reason to kickstart your journey, but do check out your underlying motivation to avoid any problems in the future.

Okay, now we know what health and wellbeing it, we know what to avoid, and we know that we have to do it for ourselves, let's check out exactly what our bodies need on a day to day basis, to be super-healthy and functioning correctly.

Discover Scientifically-Proven "Shortcuts" & "Hacks" to Lose Weight FASTER (With Very Little Effort)

For this month only, you can get Linda's best-selling & most popular book absolutely free – *Weight Loss Secrets You NEED to Know*.

Get Your FREE Copy Here:
TopFitnessAdvice.com/Bonus

Discover scientifically-proven tips to help you lose weight faster and easier than ever before. With this book, readers were able to improve their weight loss results and fitness levels. So, it's highly recommended that you get this book, especially while it's free!

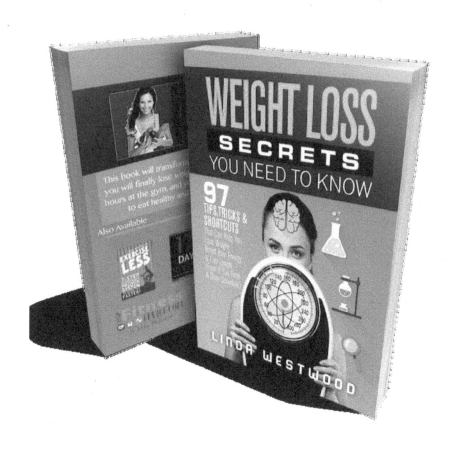

Get Your FREE Copy Here:

TopFitnessAdvice.com/Bonus

Chapter 2

The Vitamins and Minerals Essential for Good Health

We know why we need to be healthy, but how do we do it?

This book is going to give you 50 delicious recipes very shortly, which will easily allow you to pack in all the vitamins and minerals you need to function in the best possible way, but what are those essential vitamin and minerals needed for good health?

It's no good doing something unless you know why you're doing it!

Let's examine this in a little more detail.

The Vitamins and Minerals You Need

On a daily basis, your body needs the following range of vitamins and minerals:

- Vitamin A
- B vitamins
- Vitamin C (antioxidants)
- Vitamin D
- Vitamin E (antioxidants)
- Vitamin K
- Calcium
- Iodine

- Iron
- Folic Acid
- Potassium
- Zinc
- Beta-carotene
- Chromium
- Cobalt
- Copper
- Magnesium
- Manganese
- Molybdenum
- Phosphorus
- Selenium
- Sodium chloride (aka salt)
- Carbohydrates
- Protein
- Fats
- Sugar

Your body needs different amounts of all of the above, and it depends on your weight in terms of some of it for how much you need. It's impossible to give you a full overview of how much of each vitamin and mineral you need every single day, and also because daily recommended amounts are always changing.

The best advice is to consult your doctor if you have any questions about it, but packing your diet with a variation of the above every day will certainly give you a healthier lifestyle overall.

What Are Antioxidants?

If you have done any reading about health and wellbeing in the past you, will no doubt have come across the word 'antioxidant'. We're going to talk about this in many of our recipes, so it is important that we know what this term means.

Basically, antioxidants are very good things indeed. These are substances which occur in certain fruits, vegetables, chocolate and even in coffee, as well as in some of the vitamins that you need in your diet daily, such as vitamin C and E.

Antioxidants work to protect the cells within your body from damage caused by free radicals and other external factors which could potentially cause you harm. These also help your immune system to be much healthier and therefore helps you starve off illness and infection.

On the downside however, antioxidants must be balanced carefully, because if you have too many on a daily basis for a long period of time, they can turn on their heel and cause less than desirable problem, such as heart disease and certain types of cancer. Balance is everything here.

Why Fad Diets Don't Work

The fact that you have picked up this book speaks volumes. You have probably been on a diet of some kind in the past, most people have, and this diet probably didn't work for a length of time, otherwise the chances are you wouldn't be reading this book!

Whether you look at low carb diets, low calories, juice diets, and everything in-between, there is one fact that remains – the only way to become healthier, lose weight, keep it off, and to keep your body in tip top condition is to eat a balanced and varied diet, and to exercise regularly. There really is no rocket science involved!

No counting numbers, no red days and green days, no complicated maths, and no difficult meal plans – simply packing your diet with vitamins and minerals, keeping everything balanced and varied, and making sure you move as often as possible, this is all you need to change your lifestyle and become healthier, for good.

Your body is a complicated machine, it is designed to run on a careful balance, and if you throw one thing out of whack, it's going to complicate and confuse everything else too.

For instance, the Atkins Diet is based on the fact that you force your body into something called ketosis. This is basically where you flick an invisible switch in your body, and you change the usual process of burning carbs for fuel, to burning fat instead.

Of course, this means you lose weight, because you're burning the excess fat stores you have sitting around your body, but it also means that you are forcing your body to work in a different way – your body literally thinks it is going to starve, so it changes the way it functions.

Is this healthy?

There is no major evidence to suggest that the Atkins Diet is unhealthy in a serious way, when done in a careful and controlled manner, but surely simply eating things which are packed with nutrients and moving around a bit more is an easier and more healthy way to live?

There is no list of foods you can and can't eat, it's all about moderation. For instance, in this book we're going to talk about foods which can save your life, but all you need to do is incorporate them into your day, rather than only eating them and nothing else – it's not difficult, in fact it's totally do-able.

I hope that you are enjoying this book so far, and if you could spare 30 seconds, I would greatly appreciate you leaving a review on Amazon.com.

Chapter 3

Fifteen Life Saving Foods Which You Need in Your Diet

Our forthcoming recipes are all going to include a range of the superfoods we are going to talk about in this chapter. These foods are all packed with a high level of vitamins and minerals which are imperative for good health, and that means they are likely to save your life in some way!

The good news is that these diets are all ultra-flexible too, so you can easily incorporate them into your regular cooking, to give you the benefits you need for your body to function fantastically well.

Let's check out the 15 famous foods this book is based upon, and talk about why each one is so great.

Beans

Various types of beans can be used in many different recipes, and the good news is that these tiny objects are packed with countless vitamins and minerals required for good health.

In particular, beans are high in fiber, folate, and magnesium, and they can help to lower your current cholesterol level, as well as being a fantastic source of iron too. If you want more benefits, beans are also great for protein supply, whilst being low fat at the same time.

Berries

Delicious and fantastic for your health! Berries are the healthiest of all the fruits around, and they have many benefits too, including helping to guard against certain forms of cancer, and protect the liver and brain.

Your immune system is also given a major boost by chowing down on berries, because they are so packed with those antioxidants we were talking about in our previous chapter.

If you can find goji berries, these are one of the most famous superfoods of them all.

Red cabbage

You could go for kale or broccoli as an alternative if you're not the biggest fan of red cabbage, but this particular vegetable is seriously packed with those antioxidants, as well as giving you plenty of protection against certain types of cancer too.

Greens

There are countless types of greens, from broccoli to leafy greens, kale to spinach but the benefits are even more countless.

You can reduce your overall risk of developing a stroke or heart attack by around 20% if you incorporate greens into your diet. Basically, if it's green – eat it!

Mushrooms

Whilst being delicious overall and extremely flexible in terms of what you can make with them, mushrooms are a superfood in their own right.

These small fungi have nutrients which are unique to them, mainly ergothioneine, which has been linked with putting the brakes on cell death. This means you are protecting the very core of your body and its development, simply by enjoying the odd mushroom.

Flaxseeds

Ground flaxseeds can easily be added to many different recipes, but the major benefit is that they contain something called lignans. These are cancer-preventing more than perhaps anything else around.

Nuts

Who doesn't love a bowl of nuts? Whilst you should be avoiding the salted types, there are many types, such as walnuts, which are super-healthy.

By eating these regularly, you are getting a large amount of beneficial omega 3 fatty acids as well as antioxidants. All of this works to help prevent cancer development, as well as cutting your chances of having a stroke.

Turmeric

As well as being delicious as a spice, this is a serious miracle food! Turmeric contains something called curcumin which can help prevent lung and brain diseases, and is also anti-cancer too.

If you have surgery, turmeric can help you recover faster, and sufferers of rheumatoid arthritis have also found major benefit in their condition by using turmeric in their diet.

Wholegrains

If you know anything about healthy eating, you will know that wholegrains are fantastic, and are always the go-to when trying to get away from white items, such as white bread, white rice etc.

Eating wholegrains is rumoured to help you live longer, but aside from that they seriously cut the chances of heart disease, type 2 diabetes, stroke, and obesity. The other plus point is that wholegrains are so easy to find in stores these days.

Green or white tea

You've surely heard of green tea and its benefits before, but white tea is also a good option too. These help to boost your immune system and starve off illness, as well as helping you to cut your chances of developing certain types of cancer. There is some suggestion that drinking green or white tea can also cut down on blood pressure and cholesterol issues.

Oily fish

Fish like salmon, sardines, and mackerel are fantastic for your health, as well as being delicious in your recipes.

Oily fish helps to cut down the chances of developing cardiovascular disease, dementia, loss of vision due to age, and also to protect against prostate cancer in particular.

Packed with vitamin D, B, selenium, omega 3 fatty acids and proteins, this is a big-hitter food you need in your diet.

Garlic

Whether you believe in vampires or not, garlic has many uses that are nothing to do with guarding against Dracula! Not only does garlic make your food taste delicious but it also contains several vitamins and minerals, including vitamin C, B6, selenium, manganese, and plentiful antioxidants.

Pomegranate Juice

Seriously tangy and delicious, pomegranate juice in particular has been used for years in healthy beverages.

Packed with fiber, vitamins A, C, and E, as well as iron and antioxidants, pomegranate juice has been shown to be fantastic for protecting against heart disease, whilst also lowering blood pressure, protecting against certain types of cancer, and also reducing inflammation.

Beetroot

Beetroot has been used for years in alternative medicine, usually to treat skin issues, fevers, and even constipation, but beetroot is rich in iron and folate, as well as nitrates, magnesium, and antioxidants. Beetroot has also been shown to lower blood pressure, and help prevent the chances of developing dementia.

Chocolate

Now, before you get excited, putting chocolate on this list of superfoods does not mean that you can indulge in chocolate for the hell of it! We are talking about moderation here, but we are also talking about real chocolate, good quality high cocoa content chocolate.

Cocoa is shown to be a good supply for iron, manganese, magnesium, phosphorous, and zinc, as well as antioxidants. To lower stress and also help prevent certain types of cancer, chocolate is a good go-to.

These are the 15 superfoods, the foods which can save your life, that we will be basing our forthcoming recipes upon. Whilst these recipes aren't going to be totally superfood packed, they are going to be including them, in the right amounts to give you the health benefits you need.

We're going to look at breakfast, lunch, dinner, and snacks. So, without further ado, let's get cooking!

Chapter 4

Breakfast Recipes

Recipe 1 – Cereal with Goji Berries & Strawberries

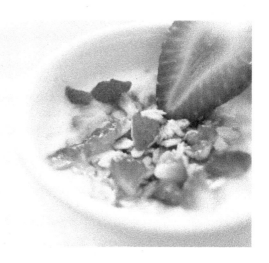

Ingredients

- Dried goji berries, 1 tablespoon
- Oat cereal (your choice), 1 serving
- Dried strawberries (diced), 0.5 cup
- Milk

Method

Place the serving of your favourite oat cereal into a bowl. Mix together the dried goji berries and the dried strawberries in a separate bowl. Now add the berries to the cereal and combine together well. Top with milk and enjoy!

Recipe 2 - Fried Egg with Spinach & Shallots

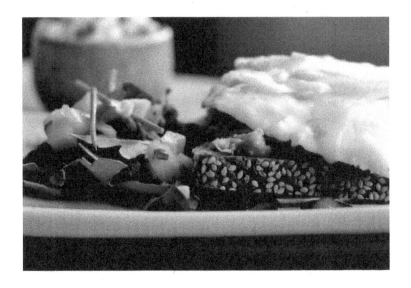

Ingredients

- Shallot x 1 (chopped)
- Coconut oil, 2 teaspoons
- Baby spinach, 1 cup
- Salt
- Pepper
- Egg, x 1

Method

Take the chopped shallot and fry it in 1 teaspoon of coconut oil, over a medium heat for around 3 minutes. Add the baby spinach. Season with salt and pepper, to your liking. Continue to cook until the spinach has wilted.

Transfer the contents of the pan to a bowl. In another pan, fry the egg in a teaspoon of coconut oil. Season with salt and pepper. Cook until it is to your liking. Serve over the spinach.

Recipe 3 – Greek Yogurt with Berries & Flaxseeds

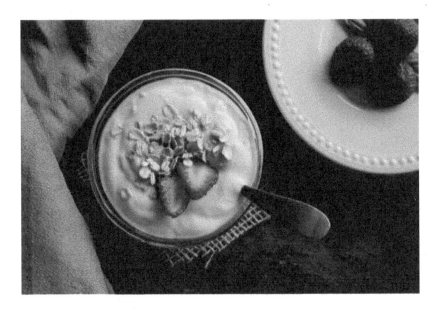

Ingredients

- Greek yoghurt, 1 cup
- Strawberries (chopped)
- Ground flax seeds, 1 tablespoon
- Honey, just a drizzle

Method

Place the cup of Greek yoghurt into a bowl and mix to separate. Add the chopped kiwi on top. Sprinkle the flax seeds over the top of the bowl. Drizzle honey over the dish, if desired.

Recipe 4 – Coconut Butter Spread with Cocoa Powder, Almonds & Honey

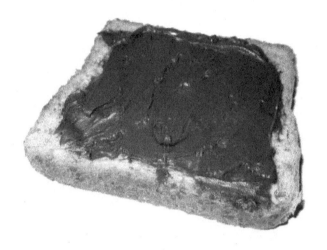

Ingredients

- Coconut butter, 1/3 cup
- Cocoa powder, 1 tablespoon
- Almonds (sliced) ¼ cup
- Honey, 1 tablespoon
- Salt (pinch)
- Wholegrain toast, 1 slice

Method

Blend together the coconut butter, cocoa powder, sliced almonds and honey in a food processor. Add a slight pinch of salt and continue to blend until smooth. Toast one piece of wholegrain bread. Spread the mixture over the bread.

Recipe 5 – Spiced Green Tea Smoothie

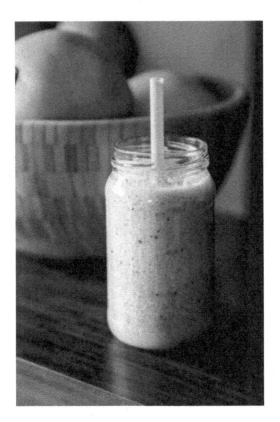

Ingredients

- Green tea (stronger the better), chilled, ¾ cup
- Cayenne pepper, 1/8 teaspoon
- Juice of 1 lemon
- Agave nectar, 2 teaspoons
- Pear (cubed), x 1
- Plain yoghurt, 2 tablespoons
- Ice cubes, x 6

Method

Place all ingredients into a food processor/blender. Blend together until smooth and combined. Pour into a serving glass and enjoy!

Recipe 6 – Cheesy Mushroom Omelette

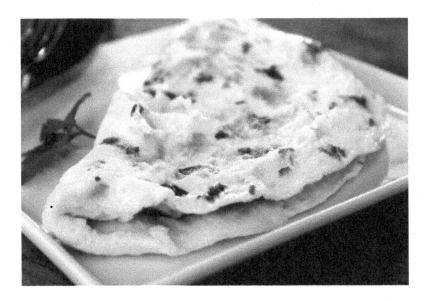

Ingredients

- Olive oil, 1 tablespoon
- Button mushrooms (sliced), 1 handful
- Cheddar cheese (grated), 25g
- Parsley leaves (chopped), a few
- Eggs (beaten), x 2

Method

Add the olive oil to a small frying pan and heat it up. Once hot, add in the mushrooms and fry for around 3 minutes, stirring occasionally. Remove the contents from the pan into a bowl. Mix in the cheese and the chopped parsley.

Put the pan back on the heat and add the beaten eggs. Cook for a minute, occasionally moving the mixture around. Over one half of the cooked omelette, spoon some of the mushrooms. Flip the other half of the omelette over, like a closed book. Leave to cook for a few more minutes and serve.

Recipe 7 – Smoky Beans on Toast

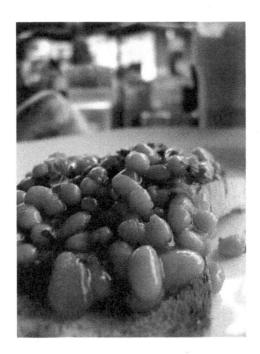

Ingredients

- Olive oil, ½ tablespoon
- Onion (sliced), ½
- Red pepper (sliced), ½
- Garlic clove, x 1
- Can of chopped tomatoes
- Smoked paprika, ½ teaspoon
- Red wine vinegar, 2 teaspoons
- Can of butter beans or chickpeas (drained)
- Sugar, ¼ teaspoon
- Wholegrain bread, 1 slice
- Parsley (chopped), a handful

Method

Heat up the oil and fry the onion and pepper for around 15 minutes. Crush half of the garlic clove and add to the frying pan. Add the tomatoes, paprika, vinegar, beans, and sugar. Mix and season with salt and pepper.

Allow the mixture to simmer for around 15 minutes, until reduced and thick. Toast the bread. Rub the other half of the garlic clove over the bread and drizzle over a little oil. Add the mixture to the toast and garnish with the parsley.

Recipe 8 – Turmeric Pancakes

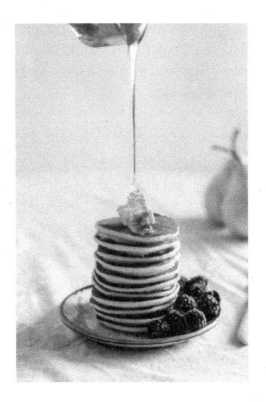

Ingredients

- Self raising flour, 200g
- Baking powder, 1 teaspoon
- Honey, 2 tablespoons
- Ground ginger, ¼ teaspoon
- Ground turmeric, ½ teaspoon
- Milk, 200ml
- Eggs, x3
- Butter, 25g

Method

Combine all ingredients (except the butter) in a bowl and mix together well. Melt the butter in a frying pan.

Add batches of the pancake mixture to the pan, in 2 tablespoon amounts, and swirl around to form circular shapes. Cook for around 2-3 minutes on each side and flip to repeat on the other side. Once all the batter has been used up, serve with your choice of topping.

Once again, thank you for reading this book, and I hope you're getting a lot of valuable information. I would greatly appreciate it if you could take 30 seconds to leave me a review for this book on Amazon.com.

Recipe 9 – Summer Porridge

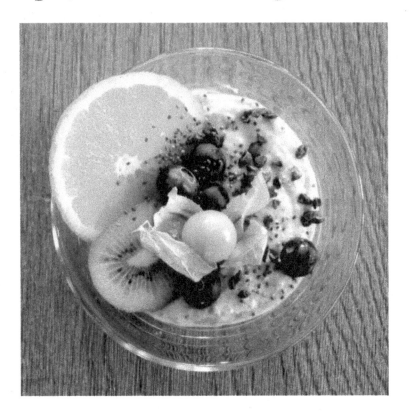

Ingredients

- Almond milk, 300ml
- Blueberries, 200g
- Maple syrup, 0.5 tablespoon
- Chia seeds, 2 tablespoons
- Jumbo oats, 100g
- Kiwi fruit (sliced), x 1
- Pomegranate seeds, 50g
- Mixed seeds, 2 teaspoons

Method

Add the milk, blueberries, and maple syrup into a blender and combine together. In a separate bowl, mix together chia seeds and the oats.

Pour the blueberry mixture over the top of the oats and mix together well. Leave for five minutes, stirring every so often. Dive the mixture between bowls. Add the fruit on top. Sprinkle over the mixed seeds.

Recipe 10 – Hash Browns with Mustard and Smoked Salmon

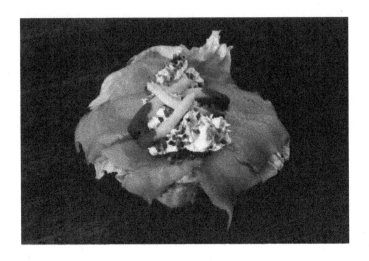

Ingredients

- Potato, x 1
- Plain flour, 1 tablespoon
- Wholegrain mustard, 1 tablespoon
- Butter, for frying
- Sunflower oil, 1 tablespoon
- Smoked salmon, x 4 slices
- Soured cream, for serving
- Chives (chopped), for garnish
- Hash browns, x 2

Method

Grate the potato over a piece of kitchen towel and press down on the towel to remove the excess water. Add the grated potato to a bowl. Add in the flour and mustard and stir together well.

Season with salt and pepper and stir again. Dive the mixture into around 8 balls and then flatten to create mini burgers. Heat the butter and oil in a large frying pan.

Add the 'burgers' to the pan and cook for around 3 minutes on each side. Add the hash browns to the plate and stack the mixture over the top. Top with a slice of smoked salmon, sourced cream and sprinkle chives over the top.

Recipe 11 – Mango and Ginger Smoothie

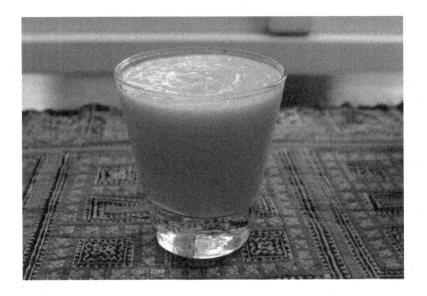

Ingredients

- Flax seed milk, 1.5 cups
- Mango (chopped), 1 cup
- Papaya, x 2 slices
- Nuts, ¼ cup
- Ginger powder, 1 teaspoons
- Turmeric, ½ teaspoons
- Chia seeds, 1 tablespoon

Method

Into a blender, add the flax seed milk, the mango, papaya and walnuts – combine. Add the ginger and turmeric and blend once more. Add the chia seeds, and blend again. Drink immediately.

Recipe 12 – Ham, Mushroom & Spinach Frittata

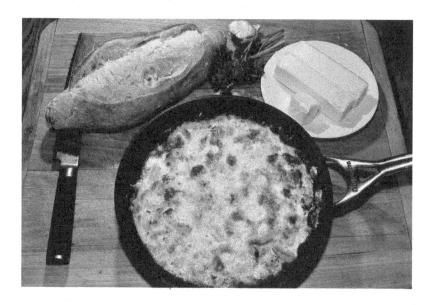

Ingredients

- Oil, 1 teaspoon
- Mushrooms (sliced), 80g
- Ham (diced), 50g
- Spinach (chopped), 80g
- Eggs (beaten), x 4
- Cheddar (grated), 1 tablespoon

Method

Heat the oil over a high heat. Fry the mushrooms for around 2 minutes. Add the ham and spinach and cook for a further minute. Season with salt and pepper.

Turn the heat down and pour the eggs over the mixture. Cook for 3 minutes, until the eggs are done. Add the cheese. Remove the pan and put under the grill for around 2 minutes.

Enjoying this book?

Check out my other best sellers!

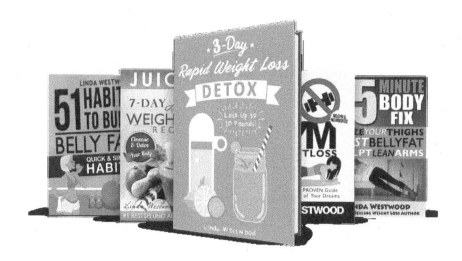

Get your next book on sale here:

TopFitnessAdvice.com/go/books

Chapter 5

Lunch Recipes

Recipe 1 – Red Lentil, Chickpea & Chilli Soup

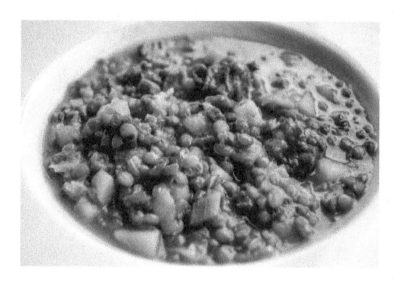

Ingredients

- Cumin seeds, 2 teaspoons
- Chilli flakes, a pinch
- Olive oil, 1 tablespoon
- Red onion (chopped), x 1
- Red split lentils, 140g
- Vegetable stock, 850ml
- Can of tomatoes, 400g
- Can of chickpeas, 200g
- Coriander (chopped), small bunch

Method

Take a large saucepan and heat it up. Add the cumin seeds and chilli flakes and fry without oil for a minute. Add the oil and the onion, cook for 5 minutes. Add the lentils, stock, and tomatoes and combine together. Bring the mixture to the boil and then all allow to simmer for 15 minutes.

Remove from the pan and add into a food processor to puree. Put the mixture ack in the pan and heat up. Season with salt and pepper and combine again. Stir in the coriander. Serve!

Recipe 2 – Smoked Mackerel Risotto

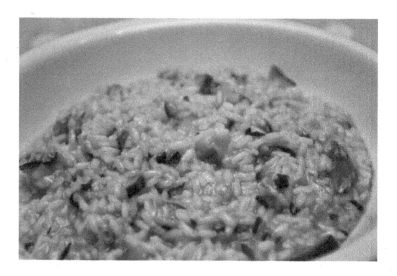

Ingredients

- Butter, 1 tablespoons
- Onion (chopped), x 1
- Risotto rice, 250g
- White wine, 100ml
- Vegetable stock, 1 litre
- Pack of smoked mackerel, x 1
- Spring onions (sliced), x 2
- Fresh spinach, 100g

Method

Melt the butter in a frying pan. Add the onion and fry for 5 minutes. Add the rice and combine until coated. Add the wine and wait for it to reduce. Add half the stock and stir well, leaving to cook for a further 10 minutes.

Add half of the remaining stock and combine once more, cooking for another 5 minutes. Add the final part of the stock and repeat. The rice should now be soft.

Peel the fish and break into pieces. Stir the fish into the rice. Add the spring onions and spinach. Cook until the spinach has wilted. Serve.

Recipe 3 – Pasta Shells with Broccoli and Anchovies

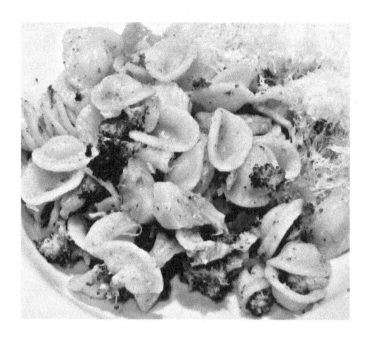

Ingredients

- Broccoli, 1 large head (cut into florets)
- Pasta shells, 400g
- Olive oil, 1 tablespoon
- Garlic cloves (sliced), x 3
- Can of anchovies (drained and chopped), x 1
- Red chilli (seeded and chopped), x 1
- Lemon, half

Method

Boil a pan of water and cook the broccoli for around 3 minutes and drain. Keep the water and cook the pasta in it. In a large pan, heat up the oil and fry the garlic. Take the garlic out of the pan and set it to one side.

Add the anchovies, chilli, and half of the water from the pasta, cooking for around 2 minutes. Add the broccoli and the lemon juice, cooking for a further minute. Add the pasta. Toss together and serve.

Recipe 4 – Warm Mackerel and Beetroot Salad

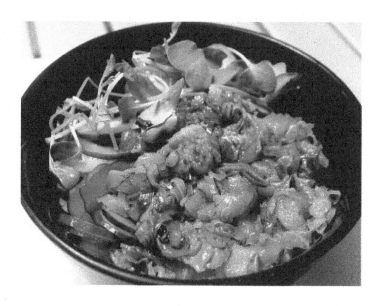

Ingredients

- Potatoes (cut into cubes), 450g
- Smoked mackerel fillets (skin removed), x 3
- Beetroot (cooked), 250g
- Mixes salad leaves, 100g bag
- Celery (sliced), x 2 sticks
- Walnut pieces, 50g
- Salad dressing, 6 tablespoons
- Creamed horseradish sauce, 2 teaspoons

Method

Boil the potatoes for around 15 minutes and drain, allowing them to cool. Take the mackerel pieces and flake. Cut the beetroot into cubes. In a separate bowl, combine the salad dressing and the horseradish sauce. Add the potatoes and toss to coat. Add the leaves, the mackerel, beetroot, celery, and the walnuts. Toss to combine and coat everything. Serve.

Recipe 5 – Garlic Bread Toasts

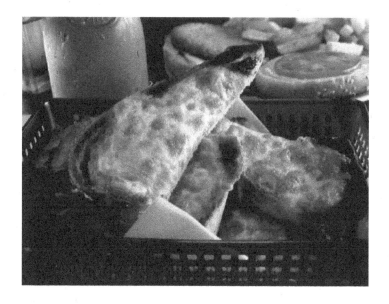

Ingredients

- Ciabatta bread loaf, x 2
- Butter, 140g
- Garlic cloves (crushed), x 6
- Parsley (chopped), a handful
- Parmesan cheese (grated), 2 tablespoons

Method

Cut the read into halves in a lengthwise manner. Toast the bread on both sides for 2 minutes – it should be very crispy. In a bowl, mix together the butter, garlic, and the parsley, to create a fragrant butter.

Spread the butter over one side of the bread. Sprinkle the parmesan over the bread. Grill for 5 minutes until everything has melted and is golden. Cut into thick wedges.

Recipe 6 – Couscous with Pine Nuts, Coriander, & Raisins

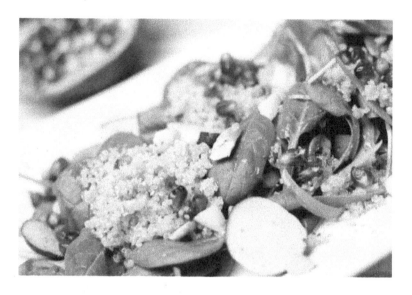

Ingredients

- Couscous, 250g
- Vegetable stock, 400ml
- Pine nuts, 75g
- Dried apricots (chopped), 50g
- Coriander leaves, 1 bunch
- Raising, 4-5 tablespoons
- The zest and juice of a lemon
- Olive oil, 5 tablespoons

Method

Take a medium bowl and add in the couscous. Pour the stock over the couscous and cover over with cling film for 5 minutes. Toast the pine nuts until they are golden. Remove the cling film and give the couscous a mix to fluff it up. Add the rest of the ingredients to the bow and combine together. Serve.

Recipe 7 – Stuffed Tomatoes

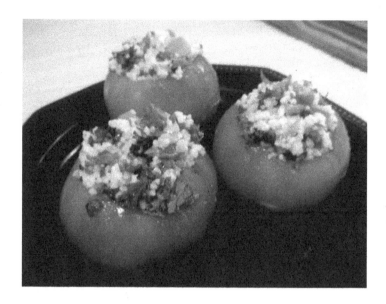

Ingredients

- Bread, x 1 slice (if it is not fresh, it's better for this recipe)
- Thyme (chopped), 1 teaspoon
- Parsley (chopped), 1 tablespoon
- Olive oil, 1 tablespoon
- Garlic clove (crushed), x 1
- Tomatoes, x 4
- Wholegrain mustard, 4 teaspoons

Method

Preheat the oven to 180 degrees C. Toast the bread and take away the crusts, before crumbling up the rest in the food processor. Add the thyme, parsley, oil, and the garlic, and mix together again.

Cut the tomatoes into halves and cover an ovenproof dish with them. On the cut side, spread over the mustard. Sprinkle some of the crumbs over the top. Place in the oven for around 20 minutes, until everything is golden and crunchy.

Recipe 8 – Green Club Sandwich

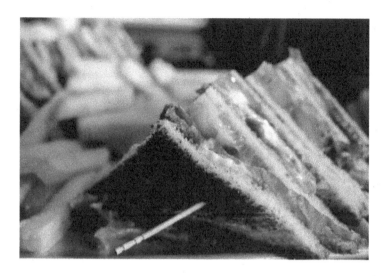

Ingredients

- Wholegrain toast, x 3 slices
- Humus, 3 tablespoons
- Avocado (sliced), x 1
- Rocket, 1 handful
- Cherry tomatoes (sliced), x 10

Method

Take the toasted bread and spread the humus over one side of each slice. On just one slice, arrange the avocado halves, the rocket, and the tomato. Season to your liking.

Add another slice of toast over the top. Add the rest of the avocado, rocket and tomato, and season. Add the final slice of bread and cut the sandwich in half.

Recipe 9 – Salmon Salad

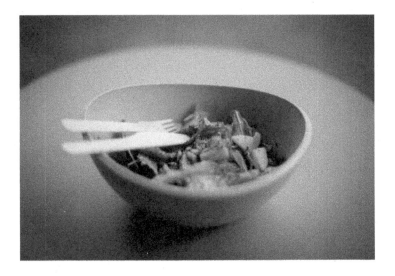

Ingredients

- Couscous, 100g
- Olive oil, 1 tablespoon
- Salmon fillets, x 2
- Broccoli (shredded), 200g
- Juice of 1 lemon
- Seeds from ½ pomegranate
- Pumpkin seeds, handful
- Watercress, handful

Method

For this recipe, you will need a steamer. Add salt and pepper to the couscous and toss with 1 teaspoon of the oil. Add boiling water to the couscous to cover for around 1cm and put to one side to soak.

Once the steamer is ready and the water is boiling, add the broccoli. Add the salmon to the upper layer of the steamer and cook for around 3 minutes. Drain the broccoli and cool. Add together the oil and lemon juice.

In a bowl, add the broccoli, pomegranate seeds, and the couscous and toss together with the lemon and oil mixture. Chop the watercress and combine with the couscous. Serve together and enjoy!

Recipe 10 – Red Cabbage, Beetroot & Apple Salad

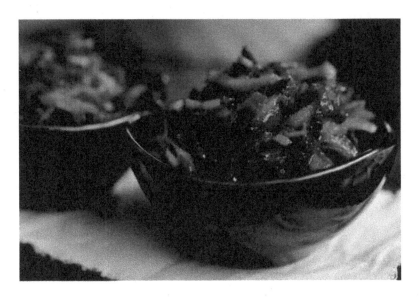

Ingredients

- Apples (sliced), x 3
- Red cabbage (sliced), 650g
- Beetroot (raw and grated), 250g
- Cider vinegar, 2 tablespoons
- Juice of half a lemon
- Olive oil, 5 tablespoons
- Pomegranate seeds, 50g
- Parsley (chopped), small bunch

Method

Into a large bowl, add the apples, red cabbage, and the beetroot, and combine. Add the vinegar, lemon juice, oil, and mix together. Pour this mixture over the cabbage bowl. Combine together well. Stir in the pomegranate and parsley. Serve.

Recipe 11 – Turmeric Scrambled Eggs

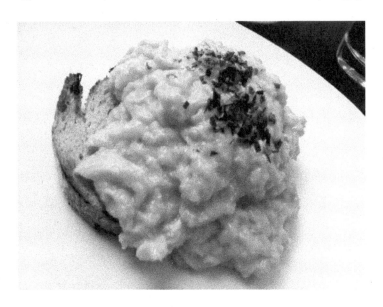

Ingredients

- Coconut oil, 1 teaspoon
- Garlic clove (chopped), ½
- Spinach leaves, 100g
- Eggs, x 4
- Coconut milk, 50ml
- Turmeric (grated), 2 teaspoons
- Wholegrain bread, x 2 slices

Method

Heat up the coconut oil over a medium heat. Fry the garlic. Add the spinach and allow to wilt. In a small bowl, whisk up the eggs with the coconut milk and the grated turmeric. Season with salt and pepper.

Add the mixture to the pan containing the spinach and cook for 5-8 minutes, stirring all the time. Serve on the bread, toasted or not.

Recipe 12 – Moroccan Chickpea Soup

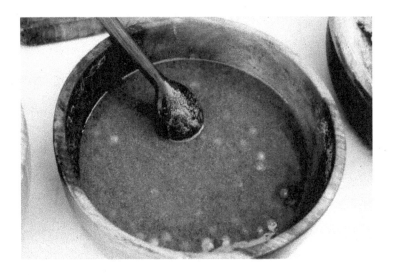

Ingredients

- Olive oil, 1 tablespoon
- Onion (chopped), x 1
- Celery (chopped), x 2 sticks
- Cumin (ground), 2 teaspoons
- Vegetable stock, 600ml
- Chopped plum tomatoes, 1 x 400g can
- Can of chickpeas (drained)
- Frozen broad beans, 100g
- The zest and juice of half a lemon
- Coriander to serve

Method

In a large pan, heat up the oil and fry the onion and celery for around 10 minutes. Add the cumin and cook for another minute, stirring occasionally. Increase the heat a little. Add the stock, tomatoes, and the chickpeas into the pan, plus black pepper. Simmer for around 8 minutes.

Add the broad beans and lemon juice, cooking for another 2 minutes. Season, and top with the coriander and a squeeze of lemon juice

Others who are considering purchasing this book would love to know what you think. If you could spare a few seconds, they would greatly appreciate reading an honest review from you. Simply visit the page on Amazon.com.

Chapter 6

Dinner Recipes

Recipe 1 – Bean Enchiladas

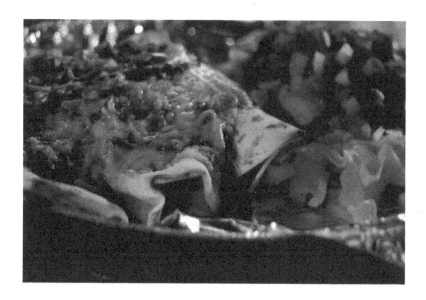

Ingredients

- Olive oil, 1 teaspoon
- Onion (chopped), x 2
- Carrots (grated), x 2
- Chilli powder, 2-3 teaspoons
- Can of chopped tomatoes, x 2
- Can of pulses (drained), x 2
- Wholemeal tortillas, x 6
- Low fat natural yoghurt, 200g
- Cheddar cheese (grated), 50g

Method

Heat up the oil in a pan. Cook the onions and the carrots until soft. Add in the chilli powder and cook for a further minute. Add the canned tomatoes and pulses and stir in, allowing to boil.

Reduce the heat and simmer for around 10 minutes, until the mixture is thick. Season, mix, and remove from the heat. Turn up your grill to high.

Take a large ovenproof serving dish and spread some of the bean mixture along the bottom. Take each tortilla and spread some of the mixture over each one, before rolling up. Place each rolled up tortillas into the dish. Pour the rest of the chilli mixture over the top of the enchiladas.

In a separate bowl, mix together the yoghurt and the cheese. Season well and combine. Spoon this over the top of the enchiladas. Place the dish under the grill for a few minutes, until golden.

Recipe 2 – Red Cabbage & Potato Hash

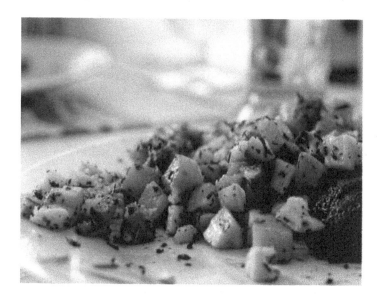

Ingredients

- Potato (diced), 800g
- Butter, 25g
- Red cabbage, 300g

Method

Boil the potatoes. Whilst the potatoes are cooking, melt the butter in a pan. Add the red cabbage to the pan and soften. Once the potatoes are cooked, drain them off.

Add to the cabbage pan. Season. Cook until the potatoes are crisp on the bottom. You can add a little more butter and continue cooking if you want your potatoes slightly crispier. Serve.

Recipe 3 – Chicken & Mushrooms

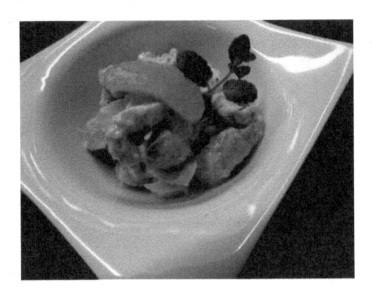

Ingredients

- Olive oil, 2 tablespoons
- Chicken thighs (boneless and skinless), 500g
- Flour
- Pancetta, 50g
- Button mushrooms, 300g
- Shallots (chopped), x 2
- Chicken stock, 250ml
- White wine vinegar, 1 tablespoon
- Frozen peas, 50g
- Parsley (chopped), small handful

Method

Heat up 1 tablespoon of oil in a large pan. Take the chicken and season it and dust with flour all over. Fry the pancetta and also the mushrooms until they are totally soft. Add the rest of the oil into the pan and cook the shallots.

Add the stock and vinegar for 2 minutes. Add the chicken to the pan, the pancetta, and the mushrooms, cooking for 15 minutes. Add in the peas and the parsley. Cook for a further 2 minutes, before serving.

Recipe 4 – Chicken Biryani

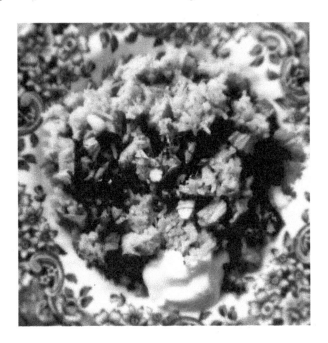

Ingredients

- Basmati rice (wholegrain if possible), 300g
- Butter, 25g
- Onion (sliced), x 1
- Bay leaf, x 1
- Cardamom pods, x 3
- Cinnamon stick, x 1
- Turmeric, 1 teaspoon
- Chicken breasts (cut into pieces), x 4
- Curry paste, x 4 tablespoons
- Raisins, 85g
- Chicken stock, 850ml
- Coriander (chopped)

Method

Take the rice and soak it in warm water, before washing. Take a saucepan and heat the butter up. Cook the onions and the bay leaf with the spices, for around 10 minutes. Add the turmeric. Add the chicken and the curry paste and cook until the smell is delicious.

Add the rice to the pan. Add the raisins. Pour in the stock. Cover the pan and bring to the boil. Once boiling, lower the heat and cook for a further 5 minutes. Turn off the heat and allow to rest for 10 minutes. Combine all the ingredients together well and add the coriander.

Recipe 5 – Sweet Mustard Salmon with Garlic Vegetables

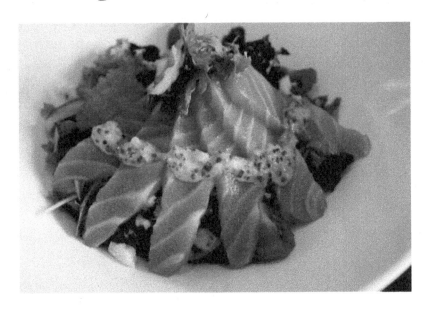

Ingredients

- New potatoes (halved), 750g
- Wholegrain mustard, 1 tablespoon
- The juice of one orange
- Honey, 2 teaspoons
- Salmon fillets (skinless and boneless), x 4
- Red peppers, x 2
- Sugar snap peas, 250g
- Olive oil, 2 tablespoons

Method

Preheat the oven to 200 degrees C. Boil the potatoes for 10 minutes. In a separate bowl, mix together the mustard, orange juice, and the honey. Coat the salmon fillets into the mixture on both sides. Cut the peppers and deseed them.

Now the potatoes are cooked, drain them and turn into an ovenproof dish. Add in the peppers and the sugar snap peas. Drizzle the dish with the oil, and season with salt and pepper, combining together. Place the salmon fillets on top. Pour over the rest of the marinade. Bake in the oven for 25 minutes.

Recipe 6 – Mackerel Fish Cakes

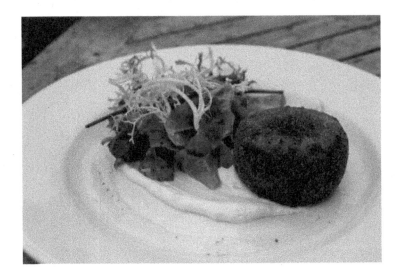

Ingredients

- Mashed potato (cold), 300g
- Spring onions (sliced), x 6
- Horseradish sauce, 1 tablespoon
- Mackerel fillets (skinned and flaked), 250g
- Plain flour, 2 tablespoons
- Egg (beaten), x 1
- Breadcrumbs, 85g

Method

Mix together the mashed potato, spring onion, horseradish, and the flaked mackerel. Take pieces of the mixture in your hands and create patties – should make around 8. Coat the fishcakes in the flour and coat on both sides. Dip the fishcakes in the beaten egg and then the breadcrumbs.

Lay on a plate and cover with cling film loosely until you are ready to cook them. If you are cooking immediately, simply fry in a little oil for 5-6 minutes on each side until golden and crunchy. Serve with a salad for a healthy main meal.

Recipe 7 – Spicy Spaghetti and Garlic Mushrooms

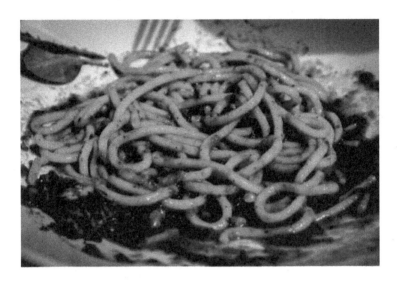

Ingredients

- Olive oil, 2 tablespoons
- Mushrooms (sliced), 250g
- Garlic clove (sliced), x 1
- Parsley, a few leaves
- Celery (chopped), x 1 stick
- Onion (chopped), x 1
- Can of chopped tomatoes, x 1
- Red chilli (chopped), ½
- Wholegrain spaghetti, 300g

Method

Heat up 1 tablespoon of the oil and fry the mushrooms for 3 minutes. Add the garlic and cook for a further minute. Tip the contents of the pan into a separate bowl and add the parsley. Return the contents of the bowl to the pan with the rest of the oil and cook for another 5 minutes.

Add the tomatoes, chilli and salt and allow to boil. Turn the heat down and simmer for 10 minutes. Cook the spaghetti and drain. Add the spaghetti to the sauce and toss.

Recipe 8 – Grilled Halloumi with Beetroot & Orange

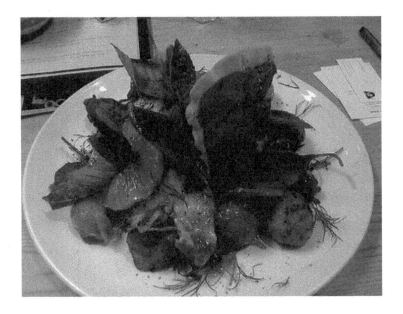

Ingredients

- Cooked beetroot, 250g
- Orange segments and juice, x 3 oranges
- White wine vinegar, 4 teaspoons
- Halloumi cheese (drained), x 2 packs
- Watercress, 100g

Method

Heat up a griddle pan to a high heat. In a bowl, mix together the beetroot, orange segments and the juice, and also the white wine vinegar, combining together well. Take the halloumi and cut it into 4 blocks per piece.

Season the halloumi with black pepper. Fry the halloumi for 2 minutes on each side, until golden. Add the watercress to the salad and toss well. Place the salad on the plate and top with the halloumi.

Recipe 9 – Black Bean Chilli

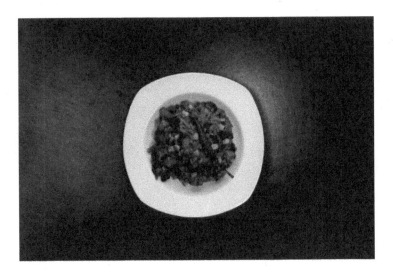

Ingredients

- Olive oil, 2 tablespoons
- Garlic cloves (chopped), x 4
- Onions (chopped), x 2
- Mild chilli powder, 3 tablespoons
- Cumin (ground), 3 tablespoons
- Cider vinegar, 3 tablespoons
- Brown sugar, 2 tablespoons
- Chopped tomatoes, x 2 cans
- Black beans (drained), x 2 cans

Method

Heat up the olive in a large pot. Cook the garlic and onions until soft. Add in the chilli powder and the cumin and continue to cook for a few more minutes.

Add the vinegar and sugar, combining well. Then add the tomatoes and season, combining again. Cook for a further 10 minutes. Add the beans and cook for another 10 minutes. Serve with rice or a salad.

Recipe 10 – Pork Chops with Fruity Red Cabbage

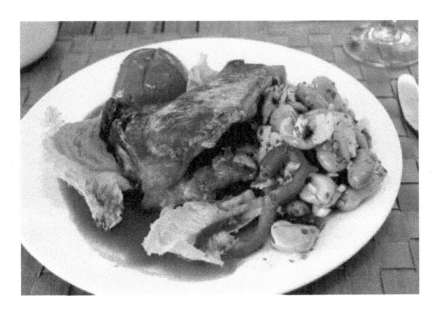

Ingredients

- Baking potatoes (cut into pieces), x 2
- Olive oil, 2 tablespoons
- Red cabbage (sliced), ½
- Onion (sliced), x 1
- Cranberry sauce, 2 tablespoons
- Apple (chopped), x 1
- Wholegrain mustard, x 2 teaspoons
- Pork chop loin, x 4

Method

Preheat the oven to 180 degrees C. Cook the potato wedges in 1 tablespoon of the oil. Heat the remaining oil in a large pan and cook the red cabbage and the onion, cooking for 5 minutes. Add in the cranberry sauce, apple, and 4 tablespoons of water.

Cover the pan over and cook for 15 minutes. Cover the top of the pork chops with the mustard and add to the tray with the potatoes. Cook for a further 5 minutes, until the meat is cooked. Serve with the cabbage mixture.

I hope you have learned something from this book so far and would greatly appreciate it if you could leave an honest review on Amazon.com.

Recipe 11 – Spicy Root & Lentil Casserole

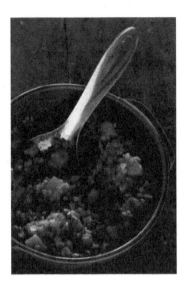

Ingredients

- Vegetable oil, 2 tablespoons
- Onion (chopped), x 1
- Garlic clove (crushed), x 2
- Potatoes (cut into chunks), 700g
- Carrot (sliced), x 4
- Parsnip (sliced), x 2
- Curry paste/powder, 2 tablespoons
- Vegetable stock, 1 litre
- Red lentils, 100g
- Coriander (chopped), small bunch

Method

Over a medium heat, heat up the oil and cook the onion and garlic for around 4 minutes. Add the potatoes, carrots and the parsnips. Turn up the heat and cook for a further 7 minutes. Add in the curry paste or powder, depending on your choice.

Add the stock and bring to the boil. Add the lentils. Cover over the pan and allow to simmer for 20 minutes. Stir in some of the coriander and combine, cooking for a further minute. Serve!

Recipe 12 – Chicken Rarebits

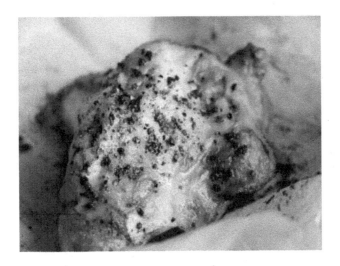

Ingredients

- Chicken fillets (boneless), x 4
- Cheddar cheese (grated), 140g
- Wholegrain mustard, 1 tablespoon
- Milk, 3 tablespoons
- Cherry tomatoes, 150g
- Broccoli, to serve

Method

Preheat the oven to 180 degrees C. Cut the chicken fillets in half. Prepare a baking dish with a little oil and lay the chicken in the dish. Mix the cheese, mustard, and milk together in a bowl.

Pour the mixture over the top of the chicken. Add the tomatoes to the dish. Cook in the oven for around half an hour. Serve with broccoli.

Recipe 13 – Fruit & Nut Butternut Squash Quinoa

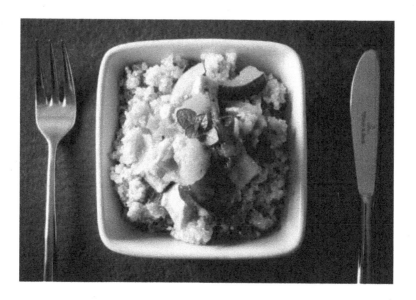

Ingredients

- Butternut squash (cubed), x 1
- Onions (sliced), x 2
- Olive oil, 2 tablespoons
- Quinoa, 200g
- Natural yoghurt, 4 tablespoons
- Tahini paste, 1 tablespoon
- Juice of 1 lemon
- Almonds (toasted), 85g
- Pistachio (shelled), 85g
- Dried apricots (sliced), x 10
- Mint leaves (chopped), a handful

Method

Preheat the oven to 200 degrees C. In a roasting tin, toss together the squash and onions, with the oil and season. Roast for half an hour, moving around occasionally. Cook the quinoa according to individual instructions and drain.

In a bowl, mix together the yoghurt, tahini, lemon juice and season. Combine the quinoa with the nuts, apricots, and mint, with a little oil. Add this to the onion and squash mixture and serve together.

Chapter 7

Snack Ideas

Recipe 1 – Chocolate & Berry Mousse Pots

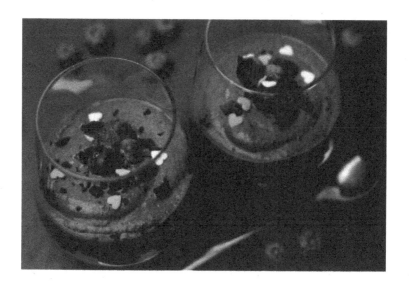

Ingredients

- Dark chocolate (grated), 75g
- Low fat yoghurt, 4 tablespoons
- Egg whites, x 2
- Caster sugar, 2 teaspoons
- Berries, 350g

Method

Melt the chocolate and then allow it to cool for 10 minutes. Once cool, stir in the yoghurt. Take the egg whites and whisk them until they form peaks. Fold the egg whites into the chocolate and yoghurt, folding in gently and keeping the air inside.

Arrange the berries into individual glasses. Divide the mixture over the top. Place in the fridge until ready to eat.

Recipe 2 – Crunchy Granola with Berries

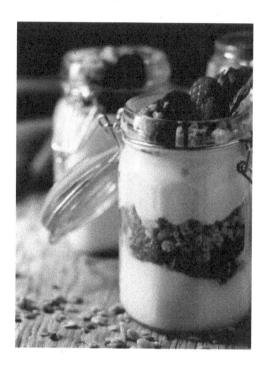

Ingredients

- Mixed nuts, 175g
- Rolled oats, 450g
- Sesame seeds, 50g
- Sunflower seeds, 50g
- Sunflower oil, 125ml
- Honey, 100ml
- Dried berries, 85g

Method

Preheat the oven to 190 degrees C. Mix the nuts with a little salt in a big bowl. Measure out the oil and pour into the bowl.

Measure out the honey and pour into the bowl. Combine together with the oats.

Prepare a large baking tray and pour the mixture on to it. Bake for 25 minutes, checking the edges aren't burning occasionally. Mix the berries with a little milk and serve with the granola mixture.

Recipe 3 – Spicy Oven Chips

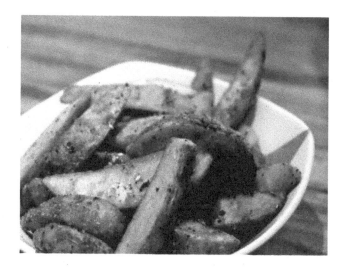

Ingredients

- Potatoes (peeled and cut into pieces), 1kg
- Turmeric, ½ teaspoon
- Sunflower oil, 3 tablespoons
- Ginger (chopped), a thumb-sized piece
- Garlic cloves (chopped), x 3
- Fennel seeds, 1 teaspoon
- Cayenne pepper, a pinch

Method

Bring the potatoes to the boil and cook with the turmeric and salt. Allow to simmer for 2-3 minutes and drain. Allow to cool – overnight is better. Preheat the oven to 180 degrees C. Take a roasting tin and prepare with 1 tablespoon of oil. Place the tin in the oven to heat up the oil.

In a bowl, add the rest of the oil with the ginger, garlic, fennel, and cayenne pepper. Now tip the potato chips into the bowl and toss well to coat all sides. Place the potatoes on the oven tray and arrange in one layer. Cook for 30 minutes, turning them over at the halfway mark.

Recipe 4 – Chocolate & Raspberry Pots

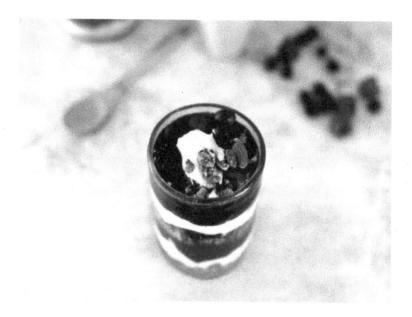

Ingredients

- Plain chocolate, 200g
- Frozen raspberries, 100g
- Greek yoghurt, 500g
- Honey, 3 tablespoons
- Chocolate sprinkles, to garnish

Method

Melt the chocolate over a low heat slowly. Allow to cool for 10 minutes. Divide the raspberries between small dishes or glasses. Mix the yoghurt and the chocolate together with the honey.

Divide the mixture over the raspberries. Refrigerate to allow the mixture to cool and form. Top with chocolate sprinkles before serving.

Recipe 5 – Acai Smoothie

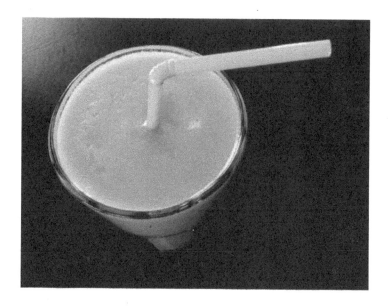

Ingredients:

- Frozen acai pulp, 100g
- Frozen pineapple, 50g
- Strawberries, 100g
- Banana, x 1
- Mango juice, 250ml
- Honey, 1 tablespoon

Method:

Blend all ingredients together using a blender. Divide into serving glasses and enjoy.

Recipe 6 – Green Tea Frozen Yoghurt

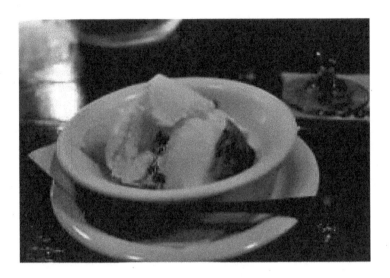

Ingredients

- Greek yoghurt, 2 x 500g pots
- Caster sugar, 200g
- Green tea matcha powder, 2 tablespoons

Method

Whisk together the yoghurt, sugar, and matcha powder until totally combined. Cover the bowl and place in the refrigerator for one hour.

Using an ice cream machine, if you have one, pour the mixture inside and follow the machine instructions. Remove from the machine and place in a container that is suitable for freezing.

Place in the freezer until you are ready to consume, waiting for at least one hours.

Recipe 7 – Fennel, Blueberry & Apple Juice

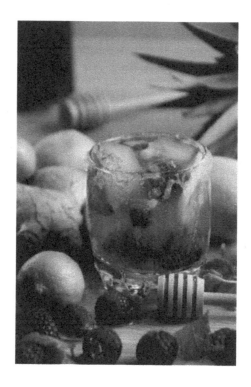

Ingredients

- Fennel bulb, x 1
- Apple (chopped), x 1
- Frozen blueberries, 85g
- Lemon juice, 1 teaspoon

Method

Cut the fennel bulb into pieces, removing the top and bottom. Place all the ingredients into the juicer and combine together. Divide between serving glasses and drink immediately.

Recipe 8 – Chilli Nuts

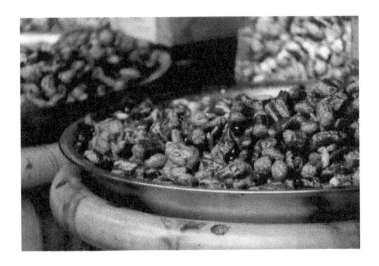

Ingredients

- Butter, 50g
- Sugar, 25g
- Cayenne pepper, ½ teaspoon
- Pecan nuts, 300g

Method

Preheat the oven to 160 degrees C. In a bowl, mix together the butter, sugar, and the cayenne pepper and combine well. Toss the pecans into the mixture and add salt if desired.

Take a baking tray and line it with baking paper. Lay the nuts on the tray. Cook for around 5 minutes. Shake the sheet and cook for another 5 minutes. Allow to cool.

Recipe 9 – Detox Salad

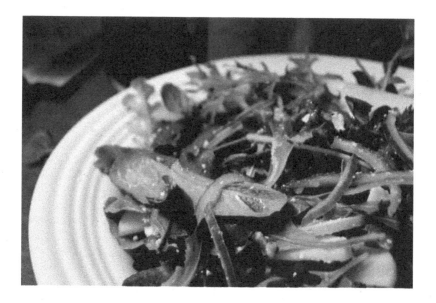

Ingredients

- Red cabbage (shredded), 350g
- Carrots (grated), x 3
- Parsley (chopped), 20g
- Apples (quartered), x 2
- Celery (sliced), x 2 sticks
- Pine nuts (toasted), 3 tablespoons
- Pumpkin seeds, 1 tablespoon
- Sunflower seeds, 2 tablespoons
- Root ginger (grated), 2 teaspoons
- Honey, 1 teaspoon
- Lemon juice, 2 tablespoons
- Olive oil, 4 tablespoons

Method

Mix all the ingredients in the bowl, apart from the juices and honey. Place the honey, lemon juice, and the oil in a separate bowl and combine together until thick. Pour the dressing over the salad and toss.

Recipe 10 – Flax & Sesame Snaps

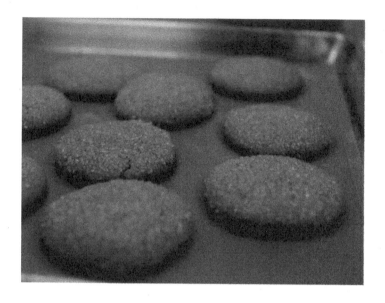

Ingredients

- Flour, 7oz
- Baking powder, ¼ teaspoon
- Butter, 5oz
- Brown sugar, 9oz
- Egg, x 1
- Vanilla extract, 1 teaspoon
- Flax seeds, 7 ½ oz
- Sesame seeds, 5 oz
- Fresh ginger (ground), 1 teaspoon

Method

Preheat the oven to 180 degrees C. Mix together the butter, sugar, egg and the vanilla, creaming really well. Mix in the flour and the baking powder and combine once more. Add the ginger and the seeds, mixing together again.

Prepare a baking tray with parchment paper. Using a teaspoon, place round sections of the batter onto the parchment paper. Bake for around 8 minutes, until browned.

Don't forget to share your thoughts on this book by leaving a review on Amazon.com. It takes just a few seconds.

Recipe 11 – Beetroot Humus

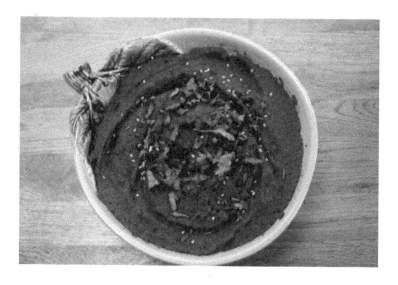

Ingredients

- Raw beetroot, 500g
- Canned chickpeas (drained), x 2
- Juice of 2 lemons
- Cumin (ground), 1 tablespoon

Method

Cook the beetroot until tender, boiling it in water for around half an hour or 40 minutes. Drain and set the beetroot aside.

Chop up the beetroot once it has cooled slightly. Place the beetroot, chickpeas, lemon juice, cumin, salt, and pepper into a food processor and combine together. Serve.

Recipe 12 – Mushrooms on Toast

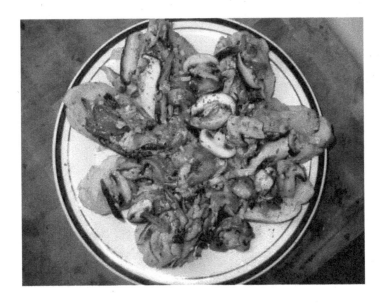

Ingredients

- Wholegrain bread, x 4 slices
- Olive oil, 1 tablespoon
- Prosciutto, x 4 slices
- Butter, small amount
- Mushrooms, 350g
- Garlic clove (crushed), x 1
- Crème fraiche, 4 tablespoons
- Parsley leaves (chopped), handful

Method

Toast the bread and set to one side. Heat up the olive oil and fry the prosciutto for 2 minutes on each side. Break the prosciutto into pieces and blot on some kitchen paper.

Add some butter to the pan and use it to cook the mushrooms for around 2 minutes. Add the garlic and the crème fraiche, and cook for another 3-5 minutes.

Stir in the parsley. Arrange the mixture on the toast and garnish with parsley.

Recipe 13 – Pomegranate Exercise Shake

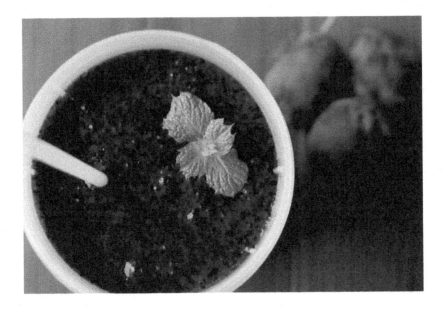

Ingredients

- Pomegranate juice, 150ml
- Soya milk, 125ml
- Banana (cubed), x 1
- Tofu, 30g
- Honey, 1 teaspoon
- Flaked almond, 1 tablespoon
- Ice cubes, a handful

Method

Blend together the pomegranate juice and soya milk, along with 2 ice cubes, until all smooth. Add in the banana, tofu, and the honey. Continue to blend until everything is combine. Pour into a serving glass. Garnish with the almonds.

Discover Scientifically-Proven "Shortcuts" & "Hacks" to Lose Weight FASTER (With Very Little Effort)

For this month only, you can get Linda's best-selling & most popular book absolutely free – *Weight Loss Secrets You NEED to Know*.

Get Your FREE Copy Here:

TopFitnessAdvice.com/Bonus

Discover scientifically-proven tips to help you lose weight faster and easier than ever before. With this book, readers were able to improve their weight loss results and fitness levels. So, it's highly recommended that you get this book, especially while it's free!

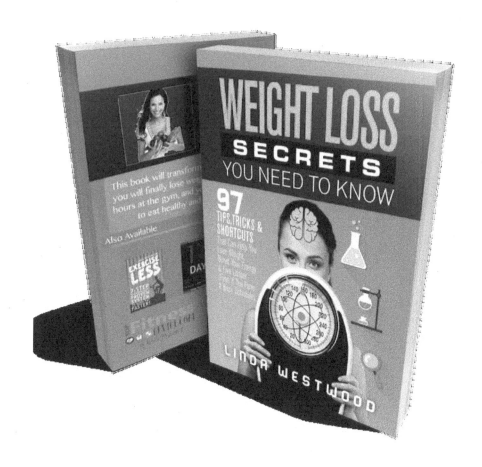

Get Your FREE Copy Here:

TopFitnessAdvice.com/Bonus

Conclusion

The idea is that by this point you are ready and raring to go, wanting to get into the kitchen and recreate some of the delicious and easy recipes we have talked about over the last few chapters.

You will also be armed with all the knowledge you need to know why you are changing your food lifestyle and incorporating these superfoods into your diet.

Remember that variation is everything, so vary these recipes and mix them up, try new things, and have fun with the foods we have mentioned, creating your own bespoke recipe ideas too.

Food is meant to be fun and delicious, a social event that we enjoy, not just something that we make in order to satisfy a bodily need for fuel and energy.

Health is important, so ditch those fad diets and look to creating healthy, sustainable habits in your life, as well as moving more often and kicking unhealthy habits and choices, to give you a much brighter future ahead of you.

Now, which recipe will you start with first?

Final Words

I would like to thank you for purchasing my book and I hope I have been able to help you and educate you on something new.

If you have enjoyed this book and would like to share your positive thoughts, could you please take 30 seconds of your time to go back and give me a review on my Amazon book page.

I greatly appreciate seeing these reviews because it helps me share my hard work.

You can leave me a review on Amazon.com.

Again, thank you and I wish you all the best!

Enjoying this book?

Check out my other best sellers!

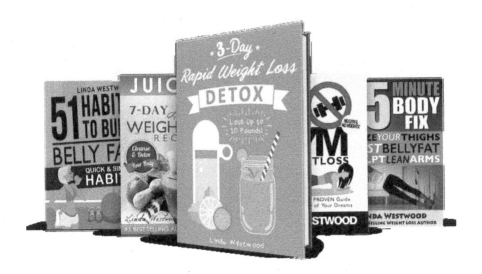

Get your next book on sale here:

TopFitnessAdvice.com/go/books